Cancer Immunoembryotherapy: A New Weapon Against Cancer

Cancer Immunoembryotherapy: A New Weapon Against Cancer

Edited by F. Columbus

Nova Science Publishers, Inc.

Art Director: Christopher Concannon
Graphics: Elenor Kallberg and Maria Ester Hawrys
Book Production: Michael Lyons, Roseann Pena,
　　　　　　　　Casey Pfalzer, June Martino,
　　　　　　　　Tammy Sauter, and Michelle Lalo
Circulation: Irene Kwartiroff, Annette Hellinger,
　　　　　　and Benjamin Fung

Library of Congress Cataloging–in–Publication Data
available upon request

ISBN 1-56072-107-3

© *1994 Nova Science Publishers, Inc.*
　6080 Jericho Turnpike, Suite 207
　Commack, New York 11725
　Tele. 516-499-3103 Fax 516-499-3146
　E Mail Novasci1@aol.com

All rights reserved. No part of this book may be reproduced, stored in a retrieval system or transmitted in any form or by any means: electronic, electrostatic, magnetic, tape, mechanical, photocopying, recording or otherwise without permission from the publishers.

Printed in the United States of America

CONTENTS

Introductory Comments	1
A Few Facts About Cancer	3
Excerpts from the Preface	17
About Professor Govallo	23
A Graphic Representation of the Immune System in Action	25
Immunoembryotherapy of Cancer—Overview	29
Detailed Description of the Book *Immunology of Pregnancy and Cancer*	33
Cancer Centers and Organizations—US	61
Cancer Centers and Organizations—Outside US	87
Action Recommendations	107
Glossary	109
Registration Form	119

INTRODUCTORY COMMENTS

This short publication is about hope. It may appear to anyone facing cancer in themselves, a relative or friend, that hope is slim. The facts are, however, that overall survival rates are increasing. In the United States, about 50% of individuals diagnosed with cancer will survive at least 5 years after diagnosis. Research efforts in this field are being carried out by some of the most brilliant medical researchers in the world. Understanding of fundamental biological processes appears very close to unlocking many secrets of nature—including cancer.

It is also hoped that the reader will learn something new from this publication including about the new and remarkable breakthrough in cancer research by Dr. Valentin Govallo. The opinions expressed on these pages are those of the publisher alone.

It is assumed that the reader of this publication has come in contact with the world of cancer. In interviews, however, we note that cancer patients frequently have little idea of what cancer is, what causes it and little comprehension of its terminology. Many do not seek a second opinion nor know the locations of various comprehensive cancer centers or are familiar with the jargon. It is hoped that this small publication will be of some help.

Frank Columbus, Publisher

A FEW FACTS ABOUT CANCER

The purpose of this section is not to attempt to deal with all the vast information available concerning cancer. It is rather to offer just a few of the basic facts. Cancer is one of the leading causes of death in the world. In the United States, for example, for anyone living into their 60's or 70's, the odds are 1 in 3 of contracting it. The actual rates tend to vary from country to country with, for some reason, a higher rate in Scotland and a lower rate in Portugal overall. Within the United States alone it is expected that about one million new cases of cancer will be diagnosed in the current year. About a third of these, or 500,000, will be "cured" through some form of treatment so that they will be alive five years from now. The other half, or 500,000 people in the U.S. alone, will not be alive five years from now. These general figures would seem to hold throughout most of the world depending, of course, on the extent or success of the various treatments. Cancer is on the rise throughout the world!

ANY NEWS?

Cancer must be presently one of the least-covered mass killers of humans in our era, if not of all time. The media is enveloped in the U.S. by other stories and articles. Research funding for cancer is inadequate. Why? Apparently because the wheel which squeaks the loudest gets greased. Cancer is old news—the word whispered; the victim pitied. But there is big news on the cancer front and lots of it—although hardly anyone knows it since our medical and investigative reporters seem to be otherwise occupied. Most newspapers across the U.S. don't even print medical sections any longer—not enough advertising to justify it, their publishers say. Should newspapers decide which news to print based on which section the automobiles, perfume makers, bra displays and wristwatch companies want to print their adds? Perhaps it is quaint to think that newspapers should be in the business of delivering the news—with the ads necessary evils. Today's newspapers, sad to say, seem to treat the news as a necessary evil—to be culled and shaped to go around the huge ads with 75% or more of every paper coupons, pictures, ads and sales leaflets. Where is the medical news? Not in the newspapers nor on television—that's for sure! Most of the medical news—certainly the news about most cancer research and its victims—is mostly left unreported!

WHAT IS CANCER?

Most people will hear or read that there really is no such as cancer. They will shake their heads in wonder as they learn that there are over 100 related diseases which are "conveniently" called cancer. Convenient for whom? This book is devoted to the similarities between cancers—not the differences. It is in the similarities that the cures reside—and where new research action is taking place. Its enough for purposes of this discussion to refer to cancer as a disease characterized by uncontrolled growth of cells that form tumors which disrupt body tissue and body functions. It is not contagious—everyone is born with the cells necessary for cancer. The question is what, when, and how and if it will be triggered. Everyone can lower his/her risk thru diet, not smoking, and electing or living under environmentally enlightened government leaders (the next one the reader may encounter could be as rare as a spotted owl!). Everyone can increase their chances for survival by being tested, paying attention to symptoms, and running, not walking, to seek appropriate medical care.

PREVENTION

The object of cancer prevention is to reduce the risk of triggering it in one's body. We can divide the methods of risk reduction into two groups: 1) Big picture cancer risk factors; and 2) Personal cancer risk factors.

Big Picture Cancer Risk Factors

It would appear clear that the biggest cancer causative factor in this category is the air, water and soil surrounding us. It is abundantly clear that our industrial leaders are: 1.) interested in their own profits first and foremost—any diseases that result are the price of "progress" (read profits!); 2.) where technology is now available ranging from scrubbers for smokestacks to low emission automobile devices—they are not used to any appreciable extent because they threaten to *lower* profits—not erase them—just lower them; 3.) government officials at all levels seem to be corrupted by personal power, perks, bribes, and the prospect of future rewards for their "services". The rare politician who is not corrupt finds himself/herself powerless before all others who are corrupt and the corruptors.

Big Picture Cancer Prevention

Nothing can be done about industry directly by the readers of this book. They have us all by the necks and we are at their mercy to a large extent. Our only recourse is to encourage industry to pay attention to the environment by purchasing products which are environmentally sensitive. If money is the object of their attention, and it clearly is—then targeted "environmental" purchasing is the only weapon.

We can change governments, however, albeit it with extraordinary difficulty. If we take it as a given that all government is corrupt, we can also assume that there is also never a shortage of candidates for office. In this observer's view, things will only improve; when mandatory term limits exist at all levels of government; and when each government body contains the same percentage of women as the general population; and when the professions of the representatives of the people are proportionate to the population as a whole—whether it be doctors, lawyers, business people, factory workers, accountants, homemakers, etc. At least in the U.S., the current system does not work and some fundamental change is necessary. The so-called representatives of the people in the U.S. seem to represent everyone's interests except those of the majority of the people. This publisher believes people would be well advised to vote for change, change, and more change at every level.

Personal Cancer Risk

The best way to reduce one's personal risk of triggering cancer in themselves is to follow the following list of do's and do not's:

Do not's

1. Do not smoke;
2. Do not take drugs;
3. Do not get exposed to excess radiation;
4. Do not sun bathe;
5. Do not have a diet heavy in dietary fat;
6. Do not get obese;
7. Do not overuse alcoholic beverages;
8. Do not assume your workplace is safe;
9. Do not eat salted of cured foods;

Here is a list of the do's to help reduce cancer risk:

1. Do eat lots green vegetables;
2. Do add fiber in your diet;
3. Do include vitamins A, C and E in your diet;
4. Do see a doctor promptly with any unusual symptoms (See Symptoms);
5. Do get tested for cancer if possible;

6. Do watch your drinking water—if in doubt purify it before consumption;
7. Do check your breasts frequently if you are a woman (remember that 1 in 8 women in the U.S. will probably get breast cancer and on Long Island, NY it may be 1 in 6);
8. Do be especially alert if your family has a history of cancer.
9. Do get frequent medical examinations.

Conclusion

We can do little short-term except scream to stop the air, water and soil from being polluted, which is then polluting all of us. It is therefore suggested that everyone try common sense and follow the do's and do not's—or be prepared to enter cancer wards. And if the reader is looking for a sign that society is interested in the slightest—it will be when cancer researchers are paid no less money for their efforts than musicians or the "average" baseball, basketball, and football players receive.

TYPES AND STAGES OF CANCER

When we discuss cancer, we must be clear that there are several types of cancer which the average person will hear about. In men most frequent types of cancer tend to be:

- lung cancer,
- stomach cancer,
- prostate cancer,
- colon cancer,
- liver cancer,
- pancreas cancer,
- rectum cancer,
- leukemia,
- cancer of the esophagus,
- bladder cancer.

In women these tend to be:

- breast cancer,
- stomach cancer,
- uterus cancer,
- colon cancer,
- liver cancer,
- lung cancer,
- cancer of the ovaries,

- cancer of the rectum,
- cancer of the pancreas,
- leukemia.

These types of cancer are listed in their rough order of mortality per type of cancer.

When one begins to talk, or think, or come into contact with cancer, one hears the work of staging or stages. It is important to know and realize what stages are all about. Usually they are divided into Stage I, II, and III. These are also referred to as Stage A, Stage B, and Stage C. There is also a Stage IV, or Stage D, which refers to certain tumors having the presence of widespread involvement of other organs, i.e., the cancer has travelled throughout the body to organs other than the organ originally containing the initial cancer. Another word or words that one runs across in "in situ", which means that it is a localized cancer. These stages of cancer and the types of cancer are very important to the individuals who are interested in this topic. The usual situation finds the patient at first stunned to learn of a cancer lurking in his or her body. One should remember however, that many cancers can be controlled or cured for years if diagnosed early.

SYMPTOMS

Here are the seven warning signs of cancer according to the American Cancer Society:

1. Change in *Bowel* or *Bladder Habits*;
2. A *Sore* that does not Heal;
3. Unusual *Bleeding* or *Discharge*;
4. Thickening of *Lump* in the Breast or Elsewhere;
5. *Indigestion* or Difficulty in *Swallowing*;
6. Obvious Change in a *Wart or Mole*;
7. Nagging *Cough or Hoarseness*.

If you have any of these signs—see your doctor now. Remember time counts!

TREATMENTS

The battle for cancer survival has continually gained new warriors. New treatments and approaches are being sought daily although the average person probably has only heard of a few of the treatments—namely radiation therapy, surgery, and chemotherapy. There are many others used on specific cancers or on an experimental basis. One also hears about all sorts of bizarre sounding cures for cancer, such as coffee enemas, and thousands of other wild-sounding treatments. There are herbs and plants and all sorts of things some of which are said to be potentially useful. The cancer patient hears about trees somewhere called Pacific Yews which are somehow used in cancer treatments. About potentially helpful drugs that for some reason the government won't approve.

Two of the most widespread fears from treatment are physical disfigurement and hair loss. The treatments for this powerful disease are of necessity potent themselves and also often cause such side effects as anemia, bleeding, constipation, diarrhea, difficulty in swallowing, dry mouth, fatigue, infection, itchy skin, loss of appetite, mouth of throat sores, nausea and vomiting, pain, respiratory problems, sexual problems, skin reactions, taste changes, and urinary tract problems. The average patient diagnosed with cancer will be told that either surgery, radiation therapy or chemotherapy is recommended and the sooner the better.

There are quacks selling cancer treatment cocktails which except for draining the cancer patients pocket seem to have little impact. The quacks never publish their results—they are supposedly too busy to do so.

IMMUNOEMBRYOTHERAPY

This publication is about a new cancer treatment called immunoembryotherapy discovered by Dr. Valentin I. Govallo and described in substantial medical detail in his new book "Immunology of Pregnancy and Cancer". This new treatment, still at the experimental stage, has been shown to be successful in previously-diagnosed terminal patients between 60–70% of the cases. The number of patients treated so far with this new therapy is, on the one hand, relatively small, and on the other hand, large enough to be persuasive that it is an effective treatment that cannot be ignored. Where this treatment goes next is dependent, to a certain extent, upon the actions of the readers of this publication. If action is demanded by the people, even the bureaucrats running everything tend to eventually do something if only to silence anyone speaking up.

Dr. Govallo's book convincingly demonstrates that there are startling medical similarities between the placenta developed during pregnancy and of a cancer tumor. Dr. Govallo has developed a new therapy based on twenty years of research using placental extracts following normal delivery (from the afterbirth), which attacks tumors. This scientific and medical book will naturally be debated, discussed, and carefully analyzed by Dr. Govallo's colleagues throughout the world. We hope that this will lead to large scale clinical tests and the treatment of large numbers of patients. It does not take a great deal of imagination to see that if the years of clinical experience accumulated by Dr. Govallo leads to anywhere near his success rate with large numbers of cancer patients, then this would be a discovery of monumental significance.

We hope that the readers of this short publication will find the text contained here to be understandable, and that they will be able to gain an understanding of this new therapy in general terms, and to take action to try to cause the therapy to be more widely used throughout the world. We present here some diagrams and sketches which we believe will explain, partially at least, the principle ideas. We recommend that the reader interested in more depth consult the book upon which these excerpts are taken as well as other books on cancer from your public library. Further in this book we are listing cancer facilities known to us at the present time, and a glossary of many of the words which one hears when coming into contact with this dreadful disease.

Remember that the keys are early detection, early treatment, positive outlook and faith.

EXCERPTS FROM THE PREFACE

We present here selected quotes from the preface of the 1992 book *Immunology of Pregnancy and Cancer* by Dr. Valentin I. Govallo.

"...When thinking of the relationship between the normal and the pathological which concerns so many people, a sad conclusion comes to mind: we were born too late because everything interesting and meaningful has already been said. The only comforting thing is that although everything has been said, not everything has been done.

More than a hundred years ago, the great German pathologist, Rudolf Virchow, mentioned that pathology had never created any new natural laws, otherwise there would be as many biologies as diseases. But biology is unique, and diseases (pathogens) only copy or pervert it; they in no way change the laws of life established by evolution.

Julius Konheim, Virchow's assistant, suggested an embryonal theory of cancer which assumed that tumors originated from embryonic cells. This theory was quickly and unanimously rejected because of the mere fact that the concept of "embryonic cell" seemed a sort of abstraction. One aspect of this theory, invisible at that time, survived: the similarities between the functional processes of cancer and the development of an embryo. Morphologists, while overlooking the implications of this theory and constantly criticizing it, nevertheless retained its theoretical basis for more than 100 years and discussed disontogenic variations of a tumor and non-tumor nature of deviations from normal embryogenesis.

Criticism of the embryonal theory was so extensive that, until recently, nobody cared to defend it. Only the facts spoke in favor of it. Gradually, mechanisms close to the embryonal type were revealed; oncogenes, growth factors and cell differentiation. Immunologists contributed to these theories, although by now Konheim's original theory was considerably modified. It turned out that malignant tumors synthesize many embryo-specific proteins; that with cancer, a heterotopic synthesis of reproductive hormones takes place; and that an organism's immune response to cancerous antigens is astonishingly similar to its response to an embryo.

Medical disciplines such as physiology, anatomy, and histology may be regarded as either normal or pathological. It is possible that in the future, such a distinction will be also recognized for immunology. Even now, allergy is often seen as the opposite to immunology. However the point is not to classify disciplines, but to understand the mechanisms for distortions of normal immune reactions. Hopefully this will suggest ways of understanding the pathogenesis of diseases and the ways to fight them. From an immunologist's point of view, it is perfectly all right to consider cancer as a "pathological embryo" which copies the normal order of immune reactions in pregnancy.

Cancer is a pathology which copies a key biological mechanism—the ability to reproduce which insures the survival of species on the level of cells and organisms. This is why cancer is so difficult to study and overcome."

"...cancer can be viewed as a perversion of the negative feedback system, while from the immunological point of view, it can be regarded as a disease of suppressory reactions in the organism.

The disharmony which was evident in the reactions of rejection (in transplantation) and suppression (cancer) require an investigation of an adequate biological model which would allow one to observe how Nature Herself is doing it. Pregnancy is such a model and is the only natural example of conflictless transplantation scheduled strictly in time."

The fact that immunological intervention can ensure the normalization of a failing pregnancy (immunization with alloantigens) and also can artificially interrupt a pregnancy (immunization with the placenta) invoked the imagination of researchers. If "peaceful coexistence" of the mother and fetus is restored artificially, then this phenomenon can lead to answers to crucial questions of transplantation immunology. The fact that reactions characteristic of the prenatal period can develop in the first trimester of pregnancy suggests solutions to certain oncological problems. Somewhere within the eternal mystery of birth and creation of new life may be hidden the secrets of the origin and possible treatment of diseases. Again, one cannot help remembering Virchow who declared in the first issue of his "Archive" that "Practical medicine is applied theoretical medicine."

The logic of the development of clinical immunology led the author to an investigation of the relationship in "mother-fetus" and "patient-tumor" systems. With a full understanding of the peculiarities of each of these fundamental biological conditions, we began to single out those features which unite the two systems.

The author is a medical doctor, so his laboratory investigations unavoidably brought him to the hospital ward. At first, his patients were the recipients of a kidney, a joint, or skin graft; then came the pregnant women experiencing multiple miscarriages, and finally, the oncological patients who had lost all hope. An immunologist is obliged to look for new solutions when all traditional methods have failed.

The structure of this book does not correspond to the chronology of studies and observations in real life. We began this research at a time when modern biotechnology did not exist, and not every clinic could provide equipment for cytofluorography, or immunoferment and radioimmune testing. Not all ideas, however, are stimulated by state-of-the-art technology."

Moscow, 1993

ABOUT PROFESSOR VALENTIN I. GOVALLO, M.D., PH.D., D.SCI.

Director, Laboratory of Clinical Immunology, Institute of Trauma and Orthopedics, Moscow. Author of 18 books, including *Immunology of Pregnancy and Cancer*, and more than 250 papers on immunology of transplantation; pregnancy and cancer published in Russian and international medical journals. Member of the Russian Academy of Medicine.

GOVALLO CANCER TEST

Dr. Govallo has developed a test involving a blood smear and analysis which is used for diagnosing malignant tumors. This test, called here the Govallo Cancer Test (GCT), is also used to determine oncogenic risk. This observer is unqualified to compare it's usefullness compared to other cancer tests. Anyone who wishes can take the GCT, and I believe it should become a standard part of every complete physical examination. Remember, the key is early detection!

A GRAPHIC REPRESENTATION OF THE IMMUNE SYSTEM IN ACTION

Immune System of a Healthy Individual (Simplified Representation)

In a healthy body there exist T-lymphocytes, B-lymphocytes, and Macrophages as well as other types of blood cells which aren't illustrated here.

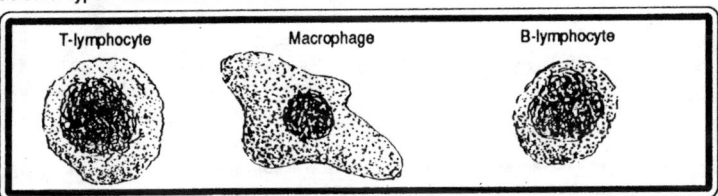

Recognition of an Intruder (Foreign Antigen)

Upon recognition of a foreign antigen II (ie. a toxin, virus, or bacteria), "virgin" B-lymphocytes divide to form memory B-lymphocytes and plasma cells which contain antibodies specific to that antigen. Upon recognition of a foreign antigen I (ie. a larger virus or infected cell), "virgin" T-lymphocytes divide to form killer T-lymphocytes and memory T-lymphocytes. Memory T-lymphocytes and memory B-lymphocytes will permit a faster and stronger immune reaction to these specific antigens if these antigens were to enter the body at a future date.

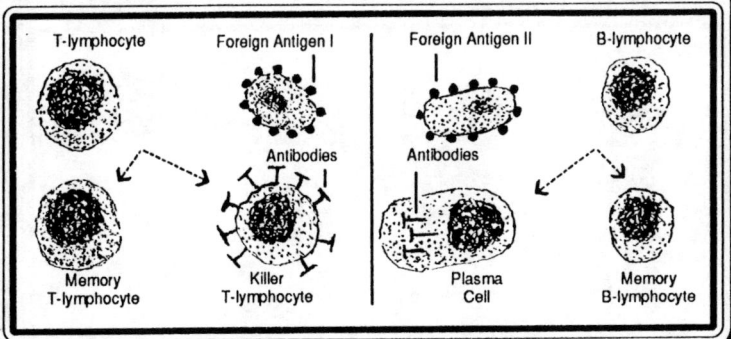

Immune System Reaction

The plasma cell releases its antibodies which attach to the foreign antigens located on the cell surface of the intruder and group these intruder cells together initiating their destruction by an existing macrophage. Killer T-lymphocytes bind to the foreign antigens located on the cell surface of the intruder which initiates the destruction of the intruder cell by the killer T-lymphocyte.

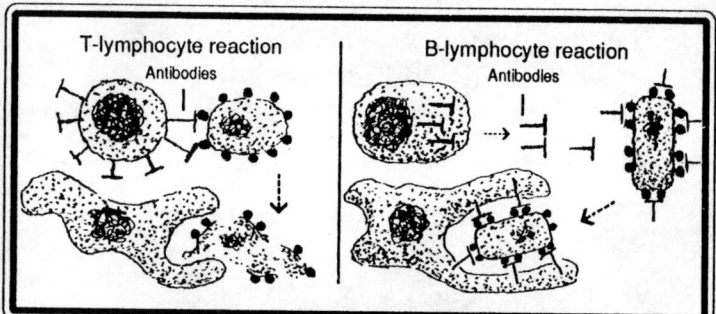

Inability of the Immune System to Fight off Cancer

Cancer cells are also foreign to the healthy body. These cells, originally part of the healthy organism have now transformed into cells which uncontrollably divide and eventually might lead to death of the organism. The immune system must initiate the destruction of these cells but cancer cells possess blocking factors which prevent their destruction by the immune system.

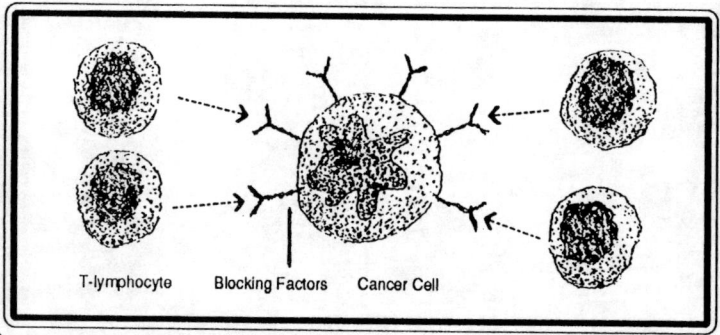

Hypothetical Deblocking Activity of Placental Extracts

The deblocking of cancer cells, illustrated on the following page, allows for the destruction of these cancer cell by the T-lymphocytes.

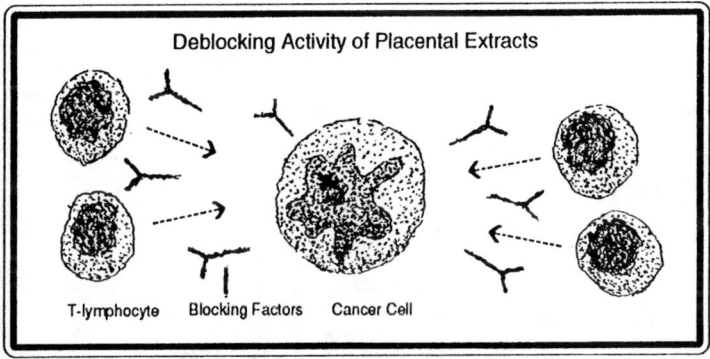

Deblocking Activity of Placental Extracts

T-lymphocyte   Blocking Factors   Cancer Cell

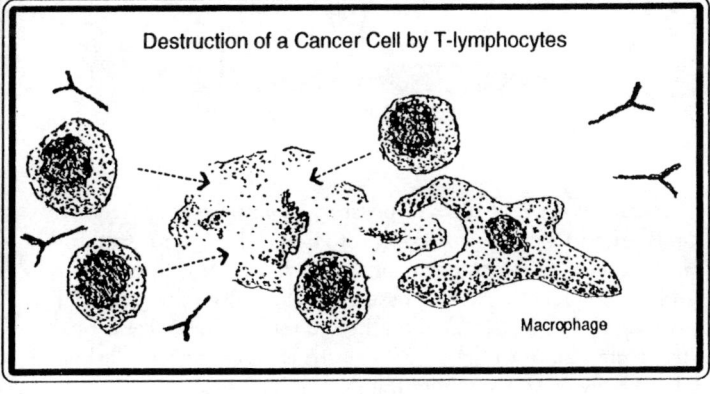

Destruction of a Cancer Cell by T-lymphocytes

Macrophage

A Hypothetical Scheme of the Deblocking Activity of Placental Extracts

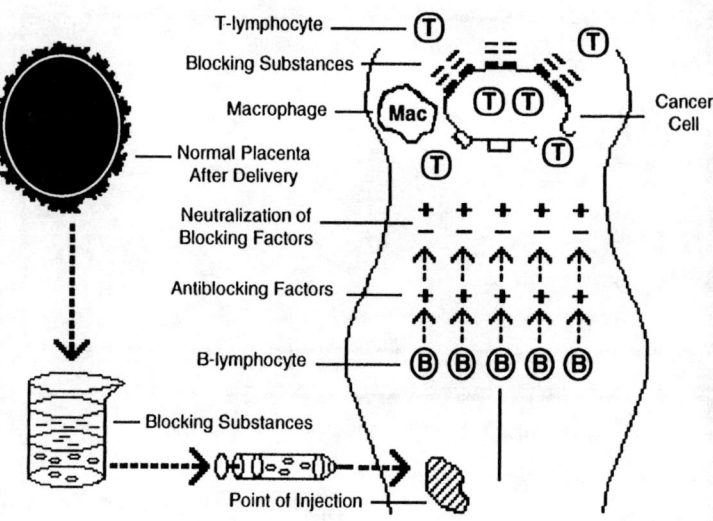

Placental extracts seem to possess properties which when administered to a cancer patient through injection, can result in the production of antiblocking factors (+) by B-lymphocytes. It is these antiblocking factors which possess the capabilty to neutralize the blocking factors (-) located on the cell membrane of cancer cells. This neutralization allows for the destruction of cancer cells by the T-lymphocytes and surrounding macrophages.

IMMUNOEMBRYOTHERAPY OF CANCER—OVERVIEW

Cancer has a dramatic immunological nature unlike any other disease. The human immunological system recognizes the presence of cancer cells, but is incapable of eliminating them. In the earliest developmental stages of cancer, the malignant cells acquire the ability to protect themselves from the host's immune system.

To understand the immunological phenomenon of cancer, it is helpful to turn to a natural model such as pregnancy. An embryo is a semi-alien entity to its mother due to the presence of the father's genes and therefore antigens. A number of mechanisms block the maternal immune system and prevent rejection of the embryo. The most important of these mechanisms is the placenta which produces powerful anti-immune effects. Maternal recognition of embryonal proteins results not in the rejection of the embryo, but in the formation of protective mechanisms which facilitate the mother-embryo interaction. If the recognition does not occur, the placental development is delayed, resulting in spontaneous abortions. In the 70s, Dr. Govallo proposed several immunotherapy treatments for complicated pregnancies. To prevent spontaneous abortions, the mothers were vaccinated with the embryo's paternal blood cells which stimulate placental growth and maintain pregnancy.

Cancer is a peculiar pseudoembryo characterized by the pathological generation of embryonal-like cells and blocking of their immunological recognition. With cancer, the strategy of immunoembryotherapy is aimed not so much at enhancing the patient's immunity as at suppressing anti-immune tactics of the tumor.

Dr. Govallo's clinical observations stratagem and laboratory research has led to the development of a placental extract vaccine which produces an anticancerous effect. This preparation is based on the proteins extracted from the placenta following normal childbirth (from the afterbirth). For 18 years, Dr. Govallo has treated patients with this preparation (vaccine) who came to him with advanced stages of breast, lung, uterine and other cancers. More than 70% of the patients have survived over 10 years with the tumors either disappeared or their growth significantly inhibited. All of the patients had been diagnosed as incurable after having undergone earlier surgery, radiation treatments, chemotherapy, separately or combined. He created the term "immunoembryotherapy" to describe the treatment. The immunoembryotherapy treatments are controlled by immunological and oncological tests. Dr. Govallo has also developed an inexpensive blood test to evaluate oncogenic risk.

DESCRIPTION OF THE BOOK *IMMUNOLOGY OF PREGNANCY AND CANCER*

We are pleased to present here the chapter titles, subtitles, and figure and table captions from Dr. Valentin Govallo's book *Immunology of Pregnancy and Cancer*. We have also included brief abstracts from each chapter as well as excerpts from the Summary.

Chapter 1.
IMMUNE SYSTEM OVERVIEW

The immune system is responsible for maintenance of homeostasis in an organism. Regulatory mechanisms of the immune system are supported by multiple cells and molecules first recognize antigens which determine tissue compatibility. The polymorphism of these antigens is extraordinarily broad for each biological species. Each organism is characterized by a specific protein formula for the antigens which are present on the surface of any cell. Immunocompetent cells recognize their own antigenic matrices and become activated when the matrices deviate from their normal status.

The human immune system includes 10^{12} lymphocytes, 20^{20} antibody molecules, and many regulatory mediators. It is a self-regulating system operating on the principles of direct and indirect, positive and negative feedback. Therefore, along with a state of specific activation, it also practices self-restriction, or immunosuppression.

1.1. ANTIGENS OF HISTOCOMPATIBILITY

Figure. Genetic scheme of MHC locus in mice (A) and humans.
Table. HLA System Nomenclature
1.1.1. MHC Antigen Expression
Conclusion

1.2. CELLULAR AND HUMORAL IMMUNE RESPONSE

Figure. Scheme of interface of immuno-competent cells.
Figure. Effect of interleukins on T and B cell differentiation.
Figure. The Structure of an IgG molecule.
Figure. Interface of an antigen and antibody 1 (Idiotype) with antibody 2 (Anti-idiotype).
Conclusion

Chapter 2.
MATERNAL RECOGNITION OF PATERNALLY-INHERITED FETAL ANTIGENS

The key issue in the establishment of normal pregnancy is the maternal recognition of foreign MHC and MHC-like antigens of the conceptus. Without this, neither the trophoblast and the placenta nor pregnancy-specific immunosuppressory mechanisms are possible. Reaction to pregnancy by immunocompetent cells of the reproductive tract and the regional lymph nodes provides a pregnant uterus with local immunity. The involvement of spleen and bone marrow in this process results in a general immunity.

Lymphokines produced by T cells and humoral antibodies synergistically affect the development of extraembryonic formations. The embryo and feto-maternal elements of the placenta produce and stimulate the formation of suppressory factors which block cytotoxic immunorejection of the fetus.

2.1. HUMORAL IMMUNE RESPONSE TO FETAL ALLOANTIGENS

Table. Women with Cytotoxic Antibodies to Paternal Lymphocytes

Conclusion

2.2. CELLULAR IMMUNE RESPONSE TO FETAL ALLOANTIGENS

LAI Technique.
- *Table.* Immunological Parameters in Blood of Pregnant Women and Healthy Donors (N = 100)
- *Table.* Hypothetical Examples of Non-Adherence Index in the LAI Test
- *Table.* Women with Positive LAI Reaction (NAI ≥ 30) to Spleen Antigen and Embryo Antigen
- *Table.* Cell Sensitization and Serum Blocking Activity of Pregnant Women
- *Table.* Sensitization and Serum Blocking Activity in Different Periods of Normal Pregnancy
- *Figure.* Mean LAI responses (non-adherence index—NAI) of pregnant women to embryo antigens and the effects of autologous serum.
- *Table.* Pregnant Women's Cell Sensitization in LAI Tests with Embryo and Adult Antigens

Conclusion

Chapter 3.
IMMUNOSUPPRESSION IN PREGNANCY

Mammalian fetuses that express paternal MHC and MHC-like antigens are not rejected by the maternal immune system. Antigen-specific and antigen-nonspecific factors have been reported to be responsible for the suppression of maternal immunity. Immunosuppression is accomplished through the joint activity of maternal lymphocytes and humoral products of fetal, decidual, and placental origin.

The highest concentration of suppressory factors occurs on the border of the feto-maternal unit. Although generalized suppression takes place, it does not cause a general maternal immunodeficiency. Humoral blocking factors and suppressory lymphocytes, induced by endogenous effects, circulate in the blood of pregnant women. The lymphocytes of pregnant women nonspecifically inhibit the recognition of allogeneic cells in MLC. In the earliest stages of pregnancy, a decrease in the percentage of small lymphocytes and an increase in the percentage of large lymphocytes is detected in blood smears.

3.1. IMMUNOSUPPRESSORY MECHANISMS IN THE PREIMPLANTATION PERIOD

3.1.1. Modulation of MHC Antigen Expression
3.1.2. Immunosuppression by Products of Semen Plasma and Sperm
3.1.3. Nonspecific Suppressory Lymphocytes and Humoral Suppressory Factor in Regional Lymph Nodes

3.1.4. Infiltration of Uterine Endometrium
by Suppressory Lymphocytes
Conclusion
3.2. DECIDUAL REACTION
Conclusion

3.3. HORMONAL REGULATION
OF IMMUNOSUPPRESSION
Conclusion

3.4. CIRCULATING LYMPHOCYTES
AND PREGNANCY DIAGNOSTICS
- *Table.* Mean Percentage of Lymphocytes in Women
- *Table.* Suppressory Lymphocytes in Blood of Pregnant Women Detected with a 3-cell MLC.
- *Table.* Functional Suppressory Lymphocytes Defected with a 3-cell MLC
- *Table.* Indices of a Pregnant Woman's Serum (SI_S), Lymphocytes (SI_l), and Serum + Lymphocytes (SI_{S+l}) in MLC
- *Figure.* The distribution of small (A) and large (B) lymphocytes in blood smears.
- *Table.* Lymphocytogram Data for Pregnant and Nonpregnant Women.

Conclusion

Chapter 4.
IMMUNOLOGY OF THE PLACENTA

The placenta is a very important immunoprotective organ which restricts the passage of alloantibodies and lymphocytes from mother to fetus. The evolution of the placenta was accompanied by increasingly intimate contact between the blood circulation systems of the mother and the fetus. It was also accompanied by a rise in the immunomodulating activity of the placenta.

Placental hormones, soluble and fixed immunosuppressory factors, and the nearly perfect impermeability of the placenta to lymphocytes and maternal antibodies make this organ a unique immunoregulatory barrier. Maximum intimacy makes it possible for oxygen, minerals, and organic substances to pass right through the placenta to the fetus. This is done without any mixing of the fetal and maternal blood circulation system. Damage of the placental barrier results in the death of the fetus and the cessation of pregnancy.

The fetal part of the placenta is not genetically identical to the maternal portion. However, paternal MHC antigens on the placenta do not serve as targets for maternal lymphocytes partly because they are masked by sialomucin, mucopolysacharides and transferrin of maternal origin, and primarialy because of the suppressory properties of the placenta itself.

Alloimmune complexes are fixed by the placenta; suppressory cells are also concentrated there. Various hormones, antigens, and lymphokines of the placenta actively inhibit antigen-recognizing functions of some T lymphocytes, and inhibits the generation of allogeneic CTL. Placental cells are capable of synthesizing remotely acting immunosuppressory substances which are present at high concentrations in the tissues of the placenta.

4.1. EVOLUTION OF THE PLACENTA

Figure. Relationship of fetus and mother (about 2 months of intrauterine development).
Figure. Schematic representation of placental types.
Figure. The structure of the human placenta.
Conclusion

4.2. ANTIGENIC STATUS OF THE PLACENTA

Conclusion

4.3. IMMUNOSUPPRESSORY PROPERTIES OF THE PLACENTA

Table. Effect of Human Placental Extracts (EVH) on Allogeneic Lymphocytes.
Conclusion

Chapter 5.
SPONTANEOUS ABORTIONS

Recurrent spontaneous abortions (RSA) are polyetiological pathologies of pregnancy; their pathogenesis is related to poor recognition of fetal alloantigens by maternal lymphocytes. As a consequence of this, lymphokines necessary for the development of the trophoblast are not produced, and blocking factors important for maintenance of pregnancy are absent.

In situations involving risk of spontaneous abortion, an additional intradermal or subcutaneous immunization of the mother with paternal blood lymphocytes normalizes pregnancy development and contributes to the birth of a healthy child. The ultimate result of this immunization is that the suppressory mechanisms of maternal immunity are stimulated. Immunological relationships in spontaneous abortions serve as a physiological model for developing methods of antiblocking therapy of cancer, since in both of these cases, the inhibition of endogenic immunosuppression takes place (See Chapters 6 and 7).

5.1 Genesis of Spontaneous Abortions
    Conclusion

5.2 IMMUNOTHERAPY OF SPONTANEOUS ABORTIONS IN CLINICAL PRACTICE

Figure. Author's Certificate of Invention. Description of Invention: A method for prevention of spontaneous abortions by means of immunological stimulation of a pregnant woman with transplants of her husband's antigens

Table. Spontaneous Abortion Immunotherapy by Paternal Skin Graft Transplants and by Injection of Paternal Lymphocytes

Table. Women Spontaneous Abortion Immunotherapy and Spontaneous Abortion Etiologies

Table. HLA-A and HLA-B Compatibility in Couples

Table. Frequency of Existence of Cell Sensitization (LAI$^+$ and Serum Immunosuppression in Women and Number of HLA Shared with Spouses

Table. Frequency of Existence of Cell Sensitization (LAI$^+$) and Serum Immunosuppression (SBA$^+$) in Women at Risk of Spontaneous Abortion Before and After Immunotherapy with Paternal Lymphocytes

Table. Occurrence of HLA Antibodies and Blocking Effects in the Serum of Women with Physiological Pregnancy and Spontaneous Abortions

5.2.1. Immunization Procedure

Table. Results of Spontaneous Abortion Immunotherapy by Injection of Paternal Lymphocytes

Figure. Mean LAI responses (non-adherence index—NAI) to embryo antigens of pregnant women's leukocytes and serum blocking autologous effect.

Table. Suppressory Lymphocytes in 3-Cell MLC of Healthy Pregnant Women and Women at Risk of Spontaneous Abortions Before and After Immunotherapy by Immunization with Paternal Lymphocytes

Table. Results of Immunotherapy by Immunizing Women at Risk of Spontaneous Abortion (SA) with Paternal Lymphocytes

Conclusion

Chapter 6.
EMBRYOLIZATION OF CANCER. IMMUNODIAGNOSTICS

Experimentation concerning immunization with embryonic tissues has revealed that expressed cross reactions between the antigens of an embryo and those of a tumor make it possible to obtain resistance to tumor growth. An increased lymphocyte sensitivity to the antigens of embryonic tissues is manifested in the earliest stage of an oncological process.

Malignant tumor growth is accompanied by the mobilization of immune suppressory factors, both cellular and humoral. The lymphocytes circulating in a patient's blood are capable of killing some tumor-like target cells *in vitro*. A positive LAI response of an oncological patient's lymphocytes to soluble embryo and tumor antigens, as well as a decrease of the small/ large lymphocyte ratio in a blood smear, are regarded as early immunological symptoms of malignization.

6.1. ANTIGENS COMMON TO EMBRYOS, TROPHOBLASTS AND TUMORS

Conclusion

6.2. CELLULAR RECOGNITION OF CANCER ANTIGENS

Table. Number and Percentage of Patients Sensitized (LAI$^+$) to Breast Cancer, Embryo and Breast Cystic Fibrosis Antigens, and Exhibiting Serum Blocking Activity (SBA)

Figure. Mean LAI responses (non-adherence index— NAI) of leukocytes from the following groups:
a) healthy women;
b) breast cancer patients in stages I–IIA before surgery;
c) breast cancer patients 0.5–2 years after surgery;
d) breast cancer patients, stage III;
e) breast cancer patients, stage IV;
f) breast cystic fibrosis patients.

Table. Number and Percentage of Patients Sensitized (LAI$^+$) to Lung Cancer, Embryo, and Tuberculoma Antigens and Exhibiting Serum Blocking Activity (SBA$^+$)

Figure. Mean LAI responses (non-adherence index—NAI) of leukocytes from the following groups:
a) healthy donors;
b) lung cancer patients in stages I–II before surgery;
c) lung cancer patients 0.5–2 years after surgery;
d) lung cancer patients, stages III–IV;
e) lung tuberculoma patients;
f) lung cystic fibrosis patients.

Figure. Mean LAI responses (non-adherence index—NAI) of leukocytes from the following groups:
a) breast cancer patients;
b) lung cancer patients;
c) osteogenic sarcoma patients. adenocarcinoma breast cancer antigens; adenocarcinoma lung cancer antigens; squamous lung cancer antigens; embryo antigens; osteogenic sarcoma antigens; giant-cell tumor antigens;

Table. Number and Percentage of Patients Sensitized (LAI$^+$) to Osteogenic Sarcoma (OS), Chondrosarcoma (ChS), Giant-Cell Tumor (GCT), and Embryo (E) Antigens, and Exhibiting Serum Blocking Activity (SBA$^+$)

Figure. Mean LAI responses (non-adherence index—NAI) of leukocytes from the following groups:
a) healthy donors;
b) osteogenic sarcoma patients;
c) chondrosarcoma patients;
d) giant-cell tumor patients. osteogenic sarcoma

antigens; chondrosarcoma antigens; giant-cell tumor antigens; embryo antigens.

Table. The Dynamics of LAI$^+$ Responses to OS and ChS Antigens by Number and Percentage with Sarcomas Before and After Surgery.

Table. Suppression by Lymphocytes and Serum from Malignant and Benign Tumors Measured in a MLC and in the Blasttransformation Reaction (BTR) with PHA.

6.2.1. Investigation of Lymphocytes-Suppressors

Table. Suppressory Blood Lymphocytes in Oncological Patients

6.2.2. Investigation of Cytolytic Functions of Lymphocytes

Figure. Cytotoxic effect of lymphocytes on target cells of human surviving fibroblasts of FL line.

Figure. Examples of the dynamics of the cytotoxic effect on human surviving fibroblasts of FL line by lymphocytes from patients with sarcomas. vertical lines: CTI for target cells (% of killed cells); horizontal line: the sequential numbers of investigation.

Table. Cytotoxic Effect (Mean CTI) on Target Cells by Lymphocytes from Healthy Donors and from Patients with Bone Tumors

Figure. The influence of autologous serum on the cytotoxic reaction of lympho-cytes of FL target cells. (the shaded area correspondes to reaction intensity); 1, 2, 3... are the sequential numbers of investigation.

Conclusion

6.3 LYMPHOCYTOGRAM AND IMMUNO-DIAGNOSTICS OF CANCER

Figure. Small lymphocytes (7.5 µm in diameter) and large lymphocytes (15 µm in diameter) in a blood smear.

Figure. Various size lymphocytes in a blood smear.

Figure. Electronogram of small (A) and large (B) lymphocytes.

Table. Lymphocyte Diameters in Blood Smears of Healthy Donors and Oncological Patients at Primary Examination

Figure. Distribution of Different Diameters of Lymphocytes inHealthy Donors and in Oncological Patients.

Table. Lymphocytes in Healthy Donors and in Patients with Tumors at Primary Examination

Table. Distribution Lymphocytes in Percoll Fractions

Table. Rosette-Formation in Purified Small and Large Lymphocytes

Table. Phenotypes of Lymphocytes from Healthy Donors and Oncological Patients

Table. Phenotypical Changes in Lymphocytes from Healthy Donors after Lymphocyte Activation by PHA *In Vitro*

Table. Characteristics of Large and Small Lymphocytes

Table. Lymphocytes of Healthy Donors and in Patients with Bone Cartilage Pathology (Absolute Numbers for a 1 mcl Sample)

Figure. The distribution of small (A) and large (B) lymphocytes in blood smears of the following groups:
a) healthy donors;
b) patients with combined trauma;
c) patients with osteomyelitis;
d) patients with sepsis;
e) patients with giant-cell tumors;
f) patients with osteo-cartilage sarcomas.
Shaded areas indicate the limits of normal values.

Table. Lymphocytes in Healthy Women and Patients with Mammary Gland Disease

Figure. Distribution of small (A) and large (B) lymphocytes in blood smears of the following groups of women:
a) healthy women;
b) breast cancer patients stages I-IIA, before operation;
c) breast cancer patients 0.5–2 years after surgery;
d) breast cancer patients stage III;
e) stage IV of breast cancer patients;
f) cystic fibrosis patients. Shaded areas indicate the limits of normal values.

Table. Immunological Indicators in Healthy Women and Women with Breast Cancer

Figure. The distribution of small (A) and large (B) lymphocytes in blood smears of the following groups:
a) healthy donors;
b) lung cancer patients stages I–II, before operation;

    c) breast cancer patients 0.5–2 years after surgery;
    d) breast cancer patients stages III–IV;
    e) tuberculosis patients;
    f) cystic fibrosis patients.

Table. Lymphocytes in Healthy Donors and Patients with Lung Pathology

Table. Immunological Indicators in Healthy Donors and Patients with Lung Disease

Table. Lymphocytes in Patients with Malignant Tumors

Figure. Dynamics of lymphocytogram indicators in oncological patients during long-term remission.

Conclusion

Figure. Description of invention: a method for diagnostics of malignant tumors in humans by means of determining the sensitization of blood lymphocytes to tumor antigens. Additionally, for a more precise diagnosis, the percentage of small lymphocytes (diameter _ 7.5 μm) is defined in the blood smear; if it decreases to 15% or lower than the norm and is accompanied by lymphocytes sensitization, a malignant tumor is diagnosed.

Chapter 7.
IMMUNOTHERAPY AND EMBRYOTHERAPY OF CANCER

The view of cancer as a disease of the entire human body, rather than a local excessive propagation of eventually invasive and metastatic cells, emerged long ago. But even today, the strategy of fighting this pathology proceeds largely from "localist" concepts. Surgery and radiation treatment are not aimed at the elimination of the major source of the disease. Chemotherapy, along with these methods, also pursues the goal of selective elimination of cells bearing a high mitotic potential, without influencing more general functions of the body. Despite the fact that oncologists themselves consider the concept of an "isolated" tumor as a figment of the imagination, the methods of treatment utilized by them are not aimed at the patient—tumor system.

Immunologists have come closer to a whole-organism approach to cancer, although so far, the results of immunotherapy of cancer have not been exceedingly impressive. Attempts to stimulate immunity to tumors similar to way immunity to infectious diseases is stimulated are not very promising, even though the immediate results can be encouraging.

Cancer is a self-sufficient pathology. It is capable of neutralizing any number of cytotoxic lymphocytes or of escaping from their specificity. It appears that more noticeable healing results can be achieved by methods which inhibit the immunosuppressory properties of the embryo-like functions of malignant cells. Immunological strategy must focus on not only augmenting the host's protective mechanisms, but also on weakening and destroying the "immunity" of the cancer. A greater emphasis should be placed on the latter, since in the early stages of disease, the immunoreactivity of the body does not suffer to a significant degree.

7.1. IMMUNOTHERAPY OF CANCER

Figure. Scheme of complex polyimmuno-therapy of a patient with osteosarcoma.

Conclusion

7.2. EMBRYOTHERAPY OF CANCER

Table. Suppressory Immunity in Pregnant Women and in Oncological Patients

Figure. Roentgenogram of Mrs. Sh. before surgery. A large, homogenous, clearly outlined shadow, 8 × 13 cm, is adjacent to the right side of the heart. Lateral to it, there are three rounded homogenous foci with clear-cut edges, with diameters of 1.5 to 2 cm (at the level of front segments of I, IV, and VII ribs). In the left lung, there are two analogous foci at the level of II and IV intercostal areas.

Figure. Roentgenogram of Mrs. Sh. three weeks after surgery and before placental extract injection. In the lower lateral section of the right lung, there is massive pleural plaque. In the left lung, the two rounded foci are still present.

Figure. Roentgenogram of Mrs. Sh. one month after therapy with placental extract. In the area of metastatic sites, in the left lung, a much smaller size shadow can be seen at the level of IVth intercostal space.

Figure. Roentgenogram of Mrs. Sh. 4 years after surgery and placental extract injection. Rounded metastatic shadows in lungs are absent.

Figure. Roentgenogram of Mrs. Sh. 7.5 years after surgery and placental extract injection. The lung tissue is normal.

Figure. Roentgenogram of Mr. Sh. before surgery. In segment IV of the right lung, there are two rounded foci, 4×6 cm and 2×2 cm, with indistinct edges.

Figure. Roentgenogram of Mr. Sh. three weeks after surgery and before placental extract injection. On the right, there is a small pleural plaque, some deformation of lung pattern and the right outline of the diaphragm.

Figure. Roentgenogram of Mr. Sh. 4 years after surgery and placental extract injection. The pleural plaque is still present on the right side, more expressed near the apex. There is aggressive growth of bone tissue in the area of rib intersection, but no indication of metastases in the lungs.

Table. Survival Rates of Oncological Patients Receiving Immunotherapy or Embryotherapy
Figure. Roentgenogram of Ms. S. In the right hip bone, a site of destruction caused by metastasis of breast cancer can be observed.
Figure. Roentgenogram of Ms. S. 10 months after placental extract injection. The destruction zone is filled with bone tissue with correctly oriented bone trabecular structure.
Figure. Roentgenogram of Ms. V. In the upper lobe of the right lung, a large rounded homogenous shadow, 5 × 6 cm, is seen. In the left lung, in the upper, medium, and lower lobes, numerous rounded shadows of a smaller size are observed. This is a case of generalized metastasizing of breast cancer into both lungs.
Figure. Roentgenogram of Ms. V. 15 months after beginning placental extract treatment. The rounded shadow in the upper part of the right lung has significantly diminished. In the left lung, the rounded shadows are not defined.
Figure. Roentgenogram of Ms. V. 19 months after the start of treatments. There are no indications of metastatic injury of the lungs. The rounded homogeneous shadows defined earlier in the right and left lungs are absent.
Figure. Hypothetical scheme of antiblocking activity of placental extract in oncological patients.

Conclusion

Selected Excerpts from the Summary

"...Progress in immunology during past decades has led to the emergence of new trends in biology and medical science. One such trend is the immunology of reproduction, the study of the role of immune factors and immunological mechanisms in the process of sexual reproduction.

Pregnancy is a unique model that can be used to study the establishment of immunity and natural "parabiosis"—the tolerance between two genetically different organisms. Pregnancy is a model of the most economical immune response to the most closely related (phylogenetically) alloantigens—MHC antigens, MHC-like antigens, and the differentiating antigens of gametes and embryos. It is a wonderful example of the harmonious combination of immune system recognition of foreign antigens and natural suppression of cytotoxic immune response. During the last decade, the immunology of reproduction has taken a giant leap forward, thanks to the development of clinical immunoprophylactic methods for spontaneous abortions and the creation of suitable experimental models.

The fact that immunological processes accompany the very beginning of life emphasizes the crucial biological importance of the immune system. The advantages of sexual, as compared to asexual, reproduction are evident: a better survival rate and the opportunity for biological perfection of heterozygotes, which is not available to homozygotes. Ever increasing antigenic polymorphism of the species inside genera warrants their biological stability. The intrauterine means of bearing offspring became the most highly developed reproductive method. All ancient instincts and the newly-developing physiological systems were called to ensure the main purpose of the living: to give life to a new, biologically better adapted, offspring."

"...In the blood smears of pregnant women, the small to large lymphocyte ratio decreases in parallel with the above-indicated characteristics. Taking into consideration the rate of development of these changes in a lymphocytogram, it is possible that this reaction is caused by the influence of reproductive hormones, and embryonic, or placental products. A considerable deficit of small lymphocytes in the lymphocytogram is observed as early as the 5th to 6th week of gestation. It can serve as a reliable diagnostic device for pregnancy. In the conditions of spontaneous abortion risk and post-delivery period, the ratio of small to large diameter lymphocytes in the lymphocytogram quickly normalizes.

In the studied forms of cancer (breast and lung) and sarcoma (bone, cartilage, blood vessels, and soft tissues) similar changes of indicators of immunity were detected: the production of the same lymphokines in the presence of both embryo antigens and antigens from histologically identical tumors; the blockage of this process *in vitro*; the accumulation of blood lymphocytes, which nonspecifically suppress an allogeneic MLC; and the reduction of the small to large lymphocyte ratio as seen in a lymphocytogram.

These observations illustrate an obvious similarity of the immunity in pregnancy and in cancer. In cancer, the perversion of the immuno-physiological reactions which help preserve the conceptus takes place. In oncological patients, cell sensitization to embryo antigens in the LAI test is more intense than in pregnancy, and the decrease of small lymphocytes is more significant. Unlike pregnancy, the indicated violations do not become normalized after surgical removal of the tumor; they recover only several years after successful cancer therapy."

"...The following known and hypothetically admissible mechanisms are immunosuppressory mechanisms common to pregnancy and cancer:

1. The fertilized ovum and stem cancer cells produce early suppressory factors affecting the closest NK cells, macrophages, and lymphocytes.
2. Hormones and lymphokines cause a nonspecific suppression–direct, or mediated via regulatory cells.
3. Both embryonic and cancerous MHC and MHC-like antigens are not immunogenic enough to cause transplantation immunity or to generate strong CTL and LAK cells.

4. TA1, TA2, and TSA types of antigens either prevent the recognition of target cells by immune lymphocytes or stimulate suppressory functions.
5. B cells synthesize humoral blocking antibodies, which independently, or together with an antigen, mask the determinants of embryonic and cancerous cells.
6. The products of extraembryonic tissues and those of malignant cells block the afferent link of immunity. The molecules of hormones, sialo-acids, transferrin, and metabolites participate in the processes of antigenic mimicry, also providing the afferent blockage of the immunity.
7. The reactive CTL receptors are blocked by anti-idiotypes.
8. Suppressory lymphocytes accumulate in regional lymph nodes, the spleen, decidual tissues, and the tumor.
9. Humoral suppressory factors having a diverse nature are present.

The idea of an immunosuppressory "shield," generated by cancer, forces us to modify approaches to the immunotherapy of cancer. It is known from experimental data that the immunization of pregnant females with embryonic cells of their extracts, when the trophoblast is intact and the placenta is not injured, is not at all dangerous to the embryo. In cases of incomplete development of the trophoblast and the placenta (primary and secondary spontaneous abortions), the immunization of pregnant women with alloantigens increases immunosuppression and prevents rejection of the fetus."

"...It became evident that in fighting cancer, deblocking therapy, aimed at the suppression of endogenic immunosuppression, must become a leading component of immunological strategy. For this therapy, we used an extract of the fetal portion of the placenta—the chorionic villi—containing a concentrate of immunosuppressory and blocking products. Even a single immunization with a large dose of placental extract achieved a reverse development of lung cancer metastases. Later on, a program of repeated placental extract injections was developed. This treatment was conducted with the immunological reactions controlled and simultaneous enhancement of functional T cells by using the extracts of embryonic thymuses. A comparative study of the blocking characteristics of different samples of placental extracts allowed the selection of the extract most suitable for a particular patient. This study was conducted using LAI tests with the blood cells of the patient and embryo antigen.

The consequences of the above-mentioned effects, termed by us as "embryotherapy," are changes of the immunoreactivity in oncological patients. In patients immunized with placental extracts, the intensity of the LAI response to embryo antigens decreased, humoral and cellular suppressory factors were eliminated from the blood, and the small/large lymphocyte ratio in the lymphocytogram gradually became normal. Clinically, in a number of cases, this process was accompanied by a reverse development of metastases and the absence of further progression of the disease. In 60% to 80% of patients with breast, lung, uterine, kidney, and other cancers, a stable remission (observed over more than 10 years of medical care) was achieved."

"...At one time, the Nobel Prize winner, Linus Pauling, suggested a concept of orthomolecular medical science, that is, treatment by use of products originating from the organism. In this case, nature itself works as a biotechnology expert. Medical science offers many examples of this phenomenon: transfusion, organ transplantation, application of antitoxic sera in infections and burns. Embryotherapy of cancer is also included in the category of orthomolecular effects. A natural biological mutual bridge must exist among human beings, and the goal of the scientist and medical doctor is to understand and control this process."

Table. Immunity Indicators in Pregnancy, Cancer and Immunotherapy

CANCER CENTERS AND ORGANIZATIONS

U.S.

**UNIVERSITY OF PUERTO RICO
PUERTO RICO CANCER CENTER**
G.P.O. Box 5067
San Juan, PR 00936
(809) 758-2525

**WORCESTER FOUNDATION
  FOR EXPERIMENTAL BIOLOGY**
Cancer Center
222 Maple Avenue
Shrewsbury, MA 01545
(617) 842-8921

DANA-FARBER CANCER INSTITUTE
44 Binney Street
Boston, MA 02115
(617) 732-3000

NEW ENGLAND DEACONESS HOSPITAL, LABORATORY OF CANCER BIOLOGY
Harvard Medical School
Department of Surgery
50 Binney Street
Boston, MA 02115
(617) 732-9876

BOSTON UNIVERSITY
HUBERT H. HUMPHREY CANCER RESEARCH CENTER (HHH-CRC)
80 East Concord Street
Boston, MA 02118
(617) 638-4173

MASSACHUSETTS INSTITUTE OF TECHNOLOGY
CENTER FOR CANCER RESEARCH
77 Massachusetts Avenue
Cambridge, MA 02139
(617) 253-6400

DANA-FARBER CANCER INSTITUTE, CANCER AND LEUKEMIA GROUP B
303 Boylston Street
Brookline, MA 02146
(617) 732-3676

CANCER RESEARCH INSTITUTE
New England Deaconess Hospital
185 Pilgrim
Boston, MA 02215
(617) 732-8016

ROGER WILLIAMS CLINICAL CANCER RESEARCH CENTER
Roger Williams General Hospital
825 Chalkstone Avenue
Providence, RI 02908
(401) 456-2070

NORRIS COTTON CANCER CENTER
Dartmouth-Hitchcock Medical Center
Hanover, NH 03756
(603) 646-5505

JOHN P. CAUFIELD TECHNOLOGY EXTENSION CENTER FOR INVESTIGATIONAL CANCER TREATMENT
1 Bruce Street
Newark, NJ 07103
(201) 456-4600

NEW YORK UNIVERSITY LABORATORY OF CANCER AND RADIOBIOLOGICAL RESEARCH
754 Brown Building
Washington Square
New York, NY 10003
(212) 598-2107

AMERICAN CANCER SOCIETY INC.
90 Park Avenue
New York, NY 10016
(800)-ACS-2345

NEW YORK UNIVERSITY KAPLAN CANCER CENTER
550 First Avenue
New York, NY 10016
(212) 340-5349

MEMORIAL SLOAN-KETTERING CANCER CENTER
1275 York Avenue
New York, NY 10021
(212) 639-2000

CANCER RESEARCH INSTITUTE, INC.
133 East 58th Street
New York, NY 10022
(212) 688-7515

COLUMBIA UNIVERSITY
COMPREHENSIVE CANCER CENTER
701 West 168th Street
New York, NY 10032
(212) 305-6921

YESHIVA UNIVERSITY
CANCER RESEARCH CENTER
Albert Einstein College of Medicine
1300 Morris Park Avenue
Bronx, NY 10461
(212) 430-2302

SYRACUSE CANCER RESEARCH INSTITUTE
600 East Genesee Street
Syracuse, NY 13202
(315) 472-6616

ROSWELL PARK MEMORIAL INSTITUTE, GRACE CANCER DRUG CENTER
666 Elm Street
Buffalo, NY 14263
(716) 845-5860

UNIVERSITY OF ROCHESTER
CANCER CENTER
601 Elmwood Avenue, Box 704
Rochester, NY 14642
(716) 275-4845

PITTSBURGH CANCER INSTITUTE
200 Meyran Avenue
Pittsburgh, PA 15213
(412) 647-2072

MERCYHURST COLLEGE CANCER RESEARCH UNIT
501 East 38th Street
Erie, PA 16546
(814) 825-0375

INSTITUTE FOR CANCER AND BLOOD DISEASES
Hahnemann University
Broad and Vine Streets
Philadelphia, PA 19102
(215) 448-8026

UNIVERSITY OF PENNSYLVANIA CANCER CENTER
3400 Spruce Street
Philadelphia, PA 19104
(215) 662-3910

FOX CHASE CANCER CENTER
7701 Burholme Avenue
Philadelphia, PA 19111
(215) 728-6900

INSTITUTE FOR CANCER RESEARCH
Fox Chase Cancer Center
7701 Burholme Avenue
Philadelphia, PA 19111
(215) 728-2491

GEORGETOWN UNIVERSITY VINCENT T. LOMBARDI CANCER RESEARCH CENTER
3800 Reservoir Avenue N.W., Podium Level
Washington, DC 20007
(202) 687-2110

AMERICAN INSTITUTE FOR CANCER RESEARCH (AICR)
1759 R Street, N.W.
Washington, DC 20009
(202) 328-7744

NATIONAL CANCER INSTITUTE
Building 31
Bethesda, MD 2025

HOWARD UNIVERSITY CANCER CENTER
2041 Georgia Avenue
Washington, DC 20060
(202) 636-7698

NATIONAL FOUNDATION FOR CANCER RESEARCH (NFRC)
7315 Wisconsin Avenue, Suite 332W
Bethesda, MD 20814
(301) 654-1250

UNIVERSITY OF MARYLAND AT BALTIMORE
UNIVERSITY OF MARYLAND CANCER CENTER
22 South Greene Street
Baltimore, MD 21201
(301) 328-5506

FREDERICK CANCER RESEARCH CENTER
P.O. Box B
Seventh Street
Frederick, MD 21701
(301) 367-7800

VIRGINIA COMMONWEALTH UNIVERSITY
MASSEY CANCER CENTER OF THE MEDICAL COLLEGE OF VIRGINIA
Box 37, MCV Station
Richmond, VA 23298
(804) 786-0449

WAKE FOREST UNIVERSITY CANCER CENTER
300 South Hawthorne Road
Winston-Salem, NC 27103
(919) 748-4464

UNIVERSITY OF NORTH CAROLINA AT CHAPEL HILL CANCER RESEARCH CENTER
Lineberger Cancer Research Center
Campus Box #7295
Chapel Hill, NC 27599-7295
(919) 966-3036

DUKE UNIVERSITY DUKE COMPREHENSIVE CANCER CENTER
P.O. Box 3814
Duke University Medical Center
Durham, NC 27710
(919) 684-3377

CHILDREN'S HOSPITAL CENTER FOR CANCER AND BLOOD DISORDERS
University of South Carolina School of Medicine
ACC 2, Area K, Richland Memorial Hospital
5 Richland Medical Park
Columbia, SC 29203
(803) 765-6484

EMORY UNIVERSITY WINSHIP CANCER CENTER
1327 Clifton Road, N.E.
Atlanta, GA 30322
(404) 248-5180

**EMORY UNIVERSITY
GEORGIA CENTER FOR CANCER STATISTICS**
1599 Clifton Road, N.E.
Atlanta, GA 30329
(404) 727-8700

POHL CANCER RESEARCH LABORATORY, INC.
Department of Chemistry and Physics
Georgia College
Milledgeville, GA 31061
(912) 453-4565

**UNIVERSITY OF MIAMI
SYLVESTER COMPREHENSIVE CANCER
 CENTER**
P.O. Box 016960 (D8-4)
School of Medicine
Miami, FL 33101
(305) 548-4800

**GOODWIN INSTITUTE FOR CANCER
 RESEARCH**
1850 Northwest 69th Avenue
Plantation, FL 33313
(305) 587-9020

H. LEE MOFFITT CANCER CENTER AND RESEARCH INSTITUTE
P.O. Box 280179
Tampa, FL 33682
(813) 972-4673

UNIVERSITY OF ALABAMA AT BIRMINGHAM COMPREHENSIVE CANCER CENTER
University Station
Birmingham, AL 35294
(205) 934-5077

CARSON-NEWMAN COLLEGE CANCER RESEARCH PROJECT
Jefferson City, TN 37760
(615) 475-9061

UNIVERSITY OF TENNESSEE MEMPHIS CANCER CENTER
3 North Dunlap Street
N327 Van Vleet Building
Memphis, TN 38163
(901) 528-5150

UNIVERSITY OF LOUISVILLE HENRY VOGT CANCER RESEARCH INSTITUTE JAMES GRAHAM BROWN CANCER CENTER
529 South Jackson Street
Louisville, KY 40292
(502) 588-6905

UNIVERSITY OF KENTUCKY CHILDREN'S CANCER STUDY GROUP
College of Medicine
Lexington, KY 40506
(606) 233-6771

McDOWELL CANCER NETWORK
800 Rose Street
Lexington, KY 40536
(606) 233-6541

UNIVERSITY OF KENTUCKY LUCILLE PARKER MARKEY CANCER CENTER
800 Rose Street
Lexington, KY 40536
(606) 257-4500

OHIO STATE UNIVERSITY COMPREHENSIVE CANCER CENTER
410 West 12th Avenue, Suite 302
Columbus, OH 43210
(614) 292-5022

HIPPLE CANCER RESEARCH CENTER
4100 South Kettering Blvd.
Dayton, OH 45439-2092
(513) 293-8508

WALTHER CANCER INSTITUTE, INC.
3202 North Meridian Street
Indianapolis, IN 46208
(317) 927-2222

PURDUE UNIVERSITY CANCER CENTER
Life Sciences Research Building
West Lafayette, IN 47907
(317) 494-9129

UNIVERSITY OF MICHIGAN KRESGE HEARING RESEARCH INSTITUTE, CANCER RESEARCH LABORATORY
1301 East Ann Street
Ann Arbor, MI 48109
(313) 764-2578

UNIVERSITY OF MICHIGAN CANCER CENTER
Cancer Research Committee
101 Simpson Drive
Box 0752
Ann Arbor, MI 48109-0752
(313) 764-0039

MEYER L. PRENTIS COMPREHENSIVE CANCER CENTER
3990 John R
Detroit, MI 48201
(313) 745-4700

MICHIGAN CANCER FOUNDATION
110 East Warren Avenue
Detroit, MI 48201
(313) 833-0710

UNIVERSITY OF IOWA CANCER CENTER
20 Medical Laboratories
Iowa City, IA 52242
(319) 335-7905

UNIVERSITY OF WISCONSIN-MADISON McARDLE LABORATORY FOR CANCER RESEARCH
Madison, WI 53706
(608) 262-2177

UNIVERSITY OF WISCONSIN CLINICAL CANCER CENTER
600 Highland Avenue
Madison, WI 53792
(608) 263-8600

UNIVERSITY OF WISCONSIN-MADISON CHILDREN'S CANCER STUDY GROUP
Department of Pediatrics
Division of Hematology/Oncology, H4/436
600 Highland Avenue
Madison, WI 53792
(608) 263-6200

UNIVERSITY OF MINNESOTA MASONIC CANCER CENTER
Division of Oncology
Box 286 University Hospital and Clinic
Harvard Street at East River Road
Minneapolis, MN 55455
(612) 624-9611

MAYO COMPREHENSIVE CANCER CENTER
200 First Street S.W.
Rochester, MN 55905
(507) 284-4718

NORTH CENTRAL CANCER TREATMENT GROUP
Operations Office
200 First Street S.W.
Rochester, MN 55905
(507) 284-8384

ILLINOIS CANCER COUNCIL COMPREHENSIVE CANCER CENTER
36 South Wabash Avenue, Suite 700
Chicago, IL 60603
(312) 346-9813

CANCER RESEARCH FOUNDATION
208 South LaSalle, Suite 721
Chicago, IL 60604
(312) 630-0055

NORTHWESTERN UNIVERSITY CANCER CENTER
303 East Chicago Avenue
Chicago, IL 60611
(312) 908-5250

RUSH CANCER CENTER
Rush-Presbyterian-St. Luke's Medical Center
1725 West Harrison Street
Chicago, IL 60612
(312) 942-6028

UNIVERSITY OF CHICAGO CANCER RESEARCH CENTER
5841 South Maryland Avenue
Chicago, IL 60637
(312) 702-6180

CANCER RESEARCH CENTER
3501 Berrywood Drive
Columbia, MO 65201
(314) 875-2255

UNIVERSITY OF KANSAS
UNIVERSITY OF KANSAS CANCER CENTER
Medical Center
Rainbow Boulevard and 39th Street
Kansas City, KS 66103
(913) 588-4700

KANSAS STATE UNIVERSITY
CENTER FOR BASIC CANCER RESEARCH
Division of Biology
Ackert Hall
Manhattan, KS 66506
(913) 532-6705

UNIVERSITY OF NEBRASKA AT OMAHA
EPPLEY INSTITUTE FOR RESEARCH IN CANCER AND ALLIED DISEASES
Medical Center
42nd and Dewey Avenue
Omaha, NE 68105
(402) 559-4238

HEREDITARY CANCER INSTITUTE
Creighton University
Omaha, NE 68178
(402) 280-2942

LINCOLN CANCER CENTER
4600 Valley Road, Suite 336
Lincoln, NE 68510
(402) 483-2827

NORTHEAST LOUISIANA UNIVERSITY CANCER RESEARCH CENTER
700 University Avenue
Monroe, LA 71209
(318) 342-2008

UNIVERSITY OF ARKANSAS ARKANSAS CANCER RESEARCH CENTER
Slot 623 UAMS
4301 West Markham
Little Rock, AR 72205
(501) 686-6000

OKLAHOMA MEDICAL RESEARCH FOUNDATION, IMMUNOLOGY AND CANCER RESEARCH PROGRAM
825 Northeast 13th Street
Oklahoma City, OK 73104
(405) 271-6673

NATALIE WARREN BRYANT CANCER CENTER
St. Francis Hospital
6161 South Yale Avenue
Tulsa, OK 74145
(918) 494-1530

STEHLIN FOUNDATION FOR CANCER RESEARCH
1315 Calhoun, Suite 1818
Houston, TX 77002
(713) 659-1336

UNIVERSITY OF TEXAS
UNIVERSITY OF TEXAS M.D. ANDERSON CANCER CENTER
Texas Medical Center
1515 Holcombe Boulevard
Houston, TX 77030
(713) 792-2121

UNIVERSITY OF TEXAS MEDICAL BRANCH AT GALVESTON CANCER CENTER
106 Basic Science Building F30
Galveston, TX 77550
(409) 761-2981

CANCER THERAPY AND RESEARCH CENTER
4450 Medical Drive
San Antonio, TX 78229
(512) 690-1111

ELEANOR ROOSEVELT INSTITUTE FOR CANCER RESEARCH
1899 Gaylord Street
Denver, CO 80206
(303) 333-4515

AMC CANCER RESEARCH CENTER
1600 Pierce Street
Denver, CO 80214
(303) 233-6501

COLORADO CANCER RESEARCH PROGRAM
Presbyterian-St. Luke's Medical Center
1719 East 19th Avenue
Denver, CO 80218
(303) 839-7788

UNIVERSITY OF UTAH ROCKY MOUNTAIN CANCER DATA SYSTEM
420 Chipeta Way #120
Salt Lake City, UT 84108
(801) 581-4307

BRIGHAM YOUNG UNIVERSITY
CANCER RESEARCH CENTER
674 WIDB
Provo, UT 84602
(801) 378-4114

ARIZONA STATE UNIVERSITY
CANCER RESEARCH INSTITUTE
Tempe, AZ 85287
(602) 965-3351

UNIVERSITY OF ARIZONA
ARIZONA CANCER CENTER
501 North Campbell Street
Tucson, AZ 85724
(602) 626-6044

UNIVERSITY OF NEW MEXICO
CANCER CENTER
900 Camino de Salud
Albuquerque, NM 87131
(505) 277-2151

UNIVERSITY OF NEVADA-RENO
ALLIE M. LEE CANCER RESEARCH
LABORATORY
157 Howard Medical Sciences
Reno, NV 89557
(702) 784-4107

UNIVERSITY OF CALIFORNIA, LOS ANGELES UCLA JONSSON COMPREHENSIVE CANCER CENTER
UCLA Medical Center
10833 LeConte Avenue
Los Angeles, CA 90024
(213) 825-5268

UNIVERSITY OF SOUTHERN CALIFORNIA LUNG DISEASE, CANCER, LYMPHOCYTES, AIR POLLUTION, AND GENERAL PATHOBIOLOGY UNIT
2011 Zonal Avenue, HMR 201
Los Angeles, CA 90033
(213) 224-7444

UNIVERSITY OF SOUTHERN CALIFORNIA COMPREHENSIVE CANCER CENTER
1441 Eastlake Avenue
P.O. Box 33800
Los Angeles, CA 90033-0800
(213) 224-6416

INSTITUTE FOR CANCER AND BLOOD RESEARCH
150 North Robertson Boulevard, #300 N
Beverly Hills, CA 90211
(213) 655-4706

CITY OF HOPE CLINICAL CANCER RESEARCH CENTER
1450 East Duarte Road
Duarte, CA 91010
(818) 357-9711

LA JOLLA CANCER RESEARCH FOUNDATION
10901 North Torrey Pines Road
La Jolla, CA 92037
(619) 455-6480

UNIVERSITY OF CALIFORNIA, SAN DIEGO CANCER CENTER
T-010
La Jolla, CA 92093
(619) 543-3608

ARMAND HAMMER CENTER FOR CANCER BIOLOGY
Salk Institute for Biological Studies
P.O. Box 85800
San Diego, CA 92138
(619) 453-4100

UNIVERSITY OF CALIFORNIA, IRVINE CANCER RESEARCH INSTITUTE
Department of Molecular Biology & Biochemistry
Irvine, CA 92717
(714) 856-5886

NORTHERN CALIFORNIA CANCER CENTER
1301 Shoreway Road, Suite 425
Belmont, CA 94002
(415) 591-4484

CHILDREN'S CANCER RESEARCH INSTITUTE
2351 Clay Street
Suite 512
San Francisco, CA 94115
(415) 923-3535

INSTITUTE OF CANCER RESEARCH
Stern Building 207
2330 Clay Street
San Francisco, CA 94115
(415) 561-1688

UNIVERSITY OF CALIFORNIA, SAN FRANCISCO CANCER RESEARCH INSTITUTE
Room 1282 Moffitt Hospital
505 Parnassus Avenue
San Francisco Medical Center
San Francisco, CA 94143-0128
(415) 476-2201

STANFORD UNIVERSITY
CANCER BIOLOGY RESEARCH LABORATORY
Stanford University Medical Center
Stanford, CA 94305
(415) 732-7312

PERLTA CANCER RESEARCH INSTITUTE
3023 Summit Street
Oakland, CA 94602
(415) 451-2369

UNIVERSITY OF CALIFORNIA, BERKELEY
CANCER RESEARCH LABORATORY
3510 Life Sciences Building
Berkeley, CA 94720
(415) 642-4711

UNIVERSITY OF HAWAII
CANCER RESEARCH CENTER OF HAWAII
1236 Lauhala Street
Honolulu, HI 96813
(808) 548-8415

FRED HUTCHINSON CANCER RESEARCH CENTER
1124 Columbia Street
Seattle, WA 98104
(206) 467-5000

CANCER CENTERS AND ORGANIZATIONS

OUSIDE OF THE U.S.

INSTITUTO DE ONCOLOGIA "ANGEL H. ROFFO"
"Angel H. Roff" Institute of Oncology
Avenida San Martin 5481
Buenos Aires, Argentina

CANCER INSTITUTE
Peter Maccallum Clinic
481 Little Lonsdale Street
Melbourne, Victoria 3000, Australia

WALTER AND ELIZA HALL INSTITUTE OF MEDICAL RESEARCH
Post Office
Royal Melbourne Hospital
Victoria 3050, Austrialia

INSTITUT JULES BORDET
1 rue Heger Bordet
1000 Brussels, Belgium

CANCER INSTITUTE
Cliniques Universitaires (St-Raphael)
Capucienenvoer 35
B-3000 Louvain, Belgium

CENTRUM VOOR GEZWELZIEKTEN
Louvain Cancer Center
Kapucihnenvoer 35
3000 Louvain, Belgium

INSTITUTO NACIONAL DE CANCER
Brazilian National Cancer Institute
Praca Cruz Vermelha 23-ZC 86
20000 Rio de Janeiro, Brazil

BRITISH COLUMBIA CANCER INSTITUTE
2656 Heather Street
Vancouver, British Columbia V5Z-3J3, Canada

MANITOBA CANCER TREATMENT AND RESEARCH FOUNDATION
700 Bannatyne Avenue
Winnipeg, Manitoba R3E 0V9, Canada

LAVAL UNIVERSITY CENTER FOR CANCER RESEARCH
Hotel-Dieu de Quebec
1 rue de l'Arsenal
Quebec, PQ, Canada G1R 2J6
(418) 691-5281

MONTREAL CANCER INSTITUTE
1560 Sherbrooke Street East
Montreal, PQ, Canada H2L 4MI
(514) 876-7078

McGILL UNIVERSITY CANCER CENTRE
3655 Drummond Street
Montreal, PQ, Canada H3G 1Y6
(514) 398-3535

CANADIAN REFERENCE CENTRE FOR CANCER PATHOLOGY
Ottawa Civic Hospital
60 Ruskin Avenue
Ottawa, ON, Canada K1Y 4M9
(613) 728-1723

McMASTER UNIVERSITY CANCER RESEARCH GROUP
Department of Pathology
Hamilton, ON, Canada L8N 3Z5
(416) 525-9140

ONTARIO CANCER TREATMENT AND RESEARCH FOUNDATION
7 Overlea Boulevard
Toronto, ON, Canada M4H 1A8
(416) 423-4240

ONTARIO CANCER INSTITUTE
500 Sherbourne Street
Toronto, ON, Canada M4X 1K9
(416) 924-0671

LONDON REGIONAL CANCER CENTRE
790 Commissioners Road East
London, ON, Canada N6A 4L6
(519) 685-8600

UNIVERSITY OF MANITOBA MANITOBA CANCER TREATMENT AND RESEARCH FOUNDATION
100 Olivia
Winnipeg, MB, Canada R3E 0V9
(204) 787-2112

TOM BAKER CANCER CENTRE
1331 29th Street, NW
Calgary, AB, Canada T2N 4N2
(403) 270-1711

CROSS CANCER INSTITUTE
11560 University Avenue
Edmonton, AB, Canada T6G 1Z2
(403) 492-8771

BRITISH COLUMBIA CANCER RESEARCH CENTRE
601 West 10th Avenue
Vancouver, BC, Canada V5Z 1L3
(604) 877-6010

CANCER CONTROL AGENCY OF BRITISH COLUMBIA DEPARTMENT OF CANCER ENDOCRINOLOGY
600 West 10th Avenue
Vancouver, BC, Canada V5Z 4E6
(604) 877-6015

J.S. MCEACHERN CANCER RESEARCH LABORATORY
Cancer Research Institute
Univ. of Alberta
Edmonton, Alta, Canada T6G 2E1

NATIONAL CANCER INSTITUTE OF CANADA
Suite 200
10 Acorn Ave
Toronto, Ontario, Canada M4V 3B1

INST. NACIONAL DEL RADIUM "DR. C.P. CORREA"
"Dr. C.P. Correa" National Radium Institute
Zanartu No 1000, Casilla No 6677
Correo No 4, Santiago de Chile, Chile

CHINESE ACADEMY OF MEDICAL SCIENCES CANCER INSTITUTE
2 Ya Pao Lu, Choa Yang District
Peking, China

INSTITUTO NACIONAL DE CANCEROLOGIA
Columbia National Cancer Institute
Calle la 9-85
Bogota, Columbia

FINSEN INSTITUTE
Strandboulevarden 49
2100 Copenhagen, Denmark

CAIRO UNIVERSITY CANCER INSTITUTE
Kasr El Aini Street
Cairo, Egypt

INSTITUTE FOR CANCER RESEARCH
17A Onslow Gardens
London, SW7 3AL, England

CHRISTIE HOSPITAL AND HOLT RADIUM INST. AND PATERSON LABS.
Withington, Manchester M20 9BX
England

CANCER SOCIETY OF FINLAND
Liisankaut 21 B9
00170 Helsinki, Finland

CENTRE PAUL PAPIN
Paul Papin Cancer Center
2 rue Moll
49036 Angers-Cedex, France

FONDATION BERGONIE, CENTRE REGIONAL ANTICANCEREUX
Bergonie Foundation Regional Cancer Center
180 rue de Saint-Genes
33076 Bordeaux Cedex, France

CENTRE REGIONAL FRANCOIS BACLESSE
Francois Baclesse Regional Cancer Center
Route de Lion sur Mer
14018 Caen Cedex, France

CENTRE GEORGE-FRANCOIS LECLERC
George-Francois Leclerc Anti-Cancer Center
1 Professor Marion Street
21034 Dijon Cedex, France

CENTRE OSCAR LAMBRET
Oscar Lambret Center
1 rue Frederic Combemale
B.P. 3569, 59020 Lille Cedex, France

INTERNATIONAL AGENCY FOR RESEARCH ON CANCER
150 cours Albert-Thomas
69372 Lyon Cedex 08, France

CENTRE LEON-BERARD
Leon Berard Center
28 rue Laennec
69373 Lyon Cedex 2, France

INSTITUT J. PAOLI-I. CALMETTES
J. Paoli-I. Calmettes Institute
232 Bd. de Sainte-Marguerite
13273 Marseilles Cedex 2, France

CENTRE REGIONAL DE LUTTE CONTRE LE CANCER
Montpellier Regional Cancer Center
Cliniques Saint Eloi
34059 Montpellier Cedex 2, France

CENTRE ANTICANCEREUX DE NANTES
Nantes Cancer Center
Quai Moncousu
44035 Nantes Cedex, France

CENTRE ANTOINE LACASSAGNE
Antoine Lacassagne Center
36 Voir-Romaine
06054 Nice Cedex, France

FONDATION CURIE - INSTITUT DU RADIUM - SECTION MED. & HOSP.
Curie Foundation - Radium Inst. - Med. & Hosp. Section
26 rue d'Ulm
75231 Paris Cedex, France

INSTITUT JEAN-GODINOT
Jean-Godinot Institute
45 rue Cognacq Jay, B.P. 171
51056 Reims Cedex, France

CENTRE REGIONAL DE LUTTE CONTRE LE CANCER DE RENNES
Rennes Regional Cancer Center
Pontachaillon
35000 Rennes, France

CENTRE HENRI-BECQUEREL
Henri-Becquerel Center
1 rue d'Amiens
76038 Rouen Cedex, France

CENTRE RENE HUGUENIN
Rene Huguenin Anti-Cancer Center
5 rue Gaston Latouche
92211 Saint-Cloud, France

CENTRE PAUL STRAUSS
Paul Strauss Regional Cancer Center
3 rue de la Poste de l'Hopital
67085 Strasbourg Cedex, France

CENTRE CLAUDIUS REGAUD
Claudius Regaud Center
11 rue Piquemil
31300 Toulouse, France

CENTRE ALEXIS VAUTRIN
Alexis Vautrin Center
R.N. 74, Brabois
54500 Vandoeuvre les Nancy, France

INSTITUT CANCER ET DIFFERCELLULAIRE
7 rue Guy Moquet
B.P. 8
94802 Villejuif, France

CENTRE TECH. POUR LE SAUT DE LA RECH. SUR CANCER
16 ave Vaillant-Couturier
B.P. 3
940801 Villejuif Cedex, France

INSTITUT GUSTAVE-ROUSSY
39 rue Camille Desmoulins
94805 Villejuif Cedex, France

ZENTRALINSTITUT FUR KREBSFORSCHUNG
Central Institute for Cancer Research
Lindenberger Weg 80
1115 Berlin-Buch, Germany

INNERE KLINIK (TUMORFORSCHUNG)
Essen Univ. Cancer Research Center
Clincal Oncology Dept.
55 Hufelandstrasse
43 Essen 1, Germany

HELLENIC ANTICANCER INSTITUTE
171 Alexandras Avenue
Athens 603, Greece

METAXAS MEMORIAL CANCER HOSPITAL
51 Botassi Street
Piraeus 30, Greece

THEAGENION MEDICAL INSTITUTE
2 Serron Street
Thessaloniki, Greece

INSTITUTO DE CANCEROLOGIA
Guatemala Cancerology Institute
6a. Av. 6-58 zona 11
Guatemala City, Guatemala

GUJARAT CANCER AND RESEARCH INSTITUTE
New Civil Hospital Campus
Asarwa, Ahmedabad 380 016, India

TATA MEMORIAL CENTRE
Ernest Borges Marg
Parel, Bombay 400 012, India

M.N.J CANCER HOSPITAL AND RADIUM INSTITUTE
11-4-720/1 Red Hills
Hyderabad 50004, India

CANCER INSTITUTE (W.I.A.)
Canal Bank Road
Adyar, Madras 600020, India

TAJ PAHLAVI CANCER INSTITUTE
University of Tehran
P.O. Box 14/1154
Tehran, Iran

SAINT ANNE'S CITY HOSPITAL FOR DISEASES OF THE SKIN AND CANCER
Northbrook Road
Dublin 6, Ireland

ST. LUKES HOSP. RADIOTHERAPY AND CLINICAL ONCOLOGY CENTRE
"Oakland", Highfield Road
Rathgar, Dublin 6, Ireland

OSPEDALE ONCOLOGICO
Cagliari Oncological Hospital
Via Jenner
Cagliari, Italy

ISTITUTO NAZIONALE PER LO STUDIO E LA CURA DEI TUMORI
National Cancer Institute
Via G. Venezian 1
20133 Milan, Italy

FOND/ SEN PASCALE-IST. PER LO STUDIO E CURA DEI TUMORI
Sen Pascale Found. Tumor Res. and Treatment Inst.
Cappella dei Cangiani Via M. Semmola
80131 Naples, Italy

SOCIETA ITALIANA DI CANCEROLOGIA
Istituto di Anatomia
Universita di Napoli
Via L. Armanni 5
80100 Naples, Italy

REGIAN ELENA INSTITUTE
Viale Regina Elena 291
00100 Rome Italy

ISTITUTO DI ONCOLOGIA DI TORINO
Turin Oncological Institute
31 via Cavour
10123 Turin, Italy

CHIBA UNIV. INST. OF PULMONARY CANCER RESEARCH
Inohana, 1-8-1
Chiba, Japan

AICHI CANCER CENTER
81-1159 Kanokoden, Tashiro-Cho Chikusa-Ku
Nogoya 464, Japan

KOKURITSU GAN CENTER
National Cancer Center
5-1-1 Tsukiji
Chuo-ku, 104 Tokyo, Japan

TOKYO UNIV. INSTITUTE OF MEDICAL SCIENCE
P.O. Takanawa
Tokyo, Japan

CANCER INSTITUTE
Kami-Ikebukuro
Toshima-ku
Tokyo 170, Japan

ZAIDANHOJIN GANNKENKYUKAI
Japanese Foundation for Cancer Research
Kami-Ikebukuro 1-37-1, Toshima-ku
Tokyo 170, Japan

YONSEI CANCER CENTER
P.O. 1010
Seoul, Korea (Rep.)

HOSPITAL DE ONCOLOGIA, C.M.N.
C.M.N. Oncological Hospital
Av. Cuauhtemoc 330
Mexico 7, D.F., Mexico

INSTITUTO NACIONAL DE CANCEROLOGIA
National Cancer Institute
Av. Ninos Heroes 151
Mexico City 7, Mexico

NEDERLANDS KANKERINST. - A. VAN LEEUWENHOEK ZIEKENHUIS
Netherlands Cancer Inst. - A. van Leeuwenhoek Hospital
Sarphatistraat 108
Amsterdam, Netherlands

NETHERLANDS CANCER INSTITUTE
Plesmanlaan 121
1066 CX Amsterdam, Netherlands

UNIVERSITAIR KANKER CENTRUM
Groningen University Cancer Center
Academisch Ziekenhuis
Oostersingel 59
Groningen, Netherlands

NORWEGIAN RADIUM HOSPITAL & NORSK HYDROS INST. FOR CANCER RESEARCH
Montebello
Oslo, Norway

INSTITUTO NACIONAL DE ENFERMEDADES NEOPLASICAS
Peruvian National Neoplastic Disease Institute
Avenida Alfonso Ugarte 825
Lima, Peru

PORTUGUESE INST. OF ONCOLOGY - FRANCISCO GENTIL
rua Prof. Lima Basto
Lisbon 4, Portugal

PUERTO RICO UNIV. COMPREHENSIVE CANCER CENTER
Univ. of Puerto Rico
P.O. Box 5067
San Juan 00936, Puerto Rico

O.F.S. INSTITUTE OF ISOTOPES AND RADIATION
National Hospital
Bloemfontein, South Africa

INSTITUTO VALENCIANO DE ONCOLOGIA
Valencia Oncology Institute
Calle Prof. Beltran Baguena 19
Valencia 9, Spain

INTERNATIONAL UNION AGAINST CANCER
3 rue du Conseil-General
1205 Geneva, Switzerland

SCHWEIZ. INST. FOR EXPER. KREBSFORSCHUNG
Ch. des Boveresses 155
1066 Epalinges S.
Lausanne, Switzerland

INSTITUTO DE RADIOLOGIA
Montevideo Institute of Radiology
Bulevar Artigas No. 1550
Montevideo, Uruguay

HOSPITAL ONCOLOGICO "PADRE MACHADO"
"Padre Machado" Oncological Hospital
Calle El Degredo
Los Castanos El Cementerio
Caracas DF, Venezuela

ACTION RECOMMENDATIONS

This observer has studied the data, seen the patients, read the book, visited the laboratory, speaks the language, and knows the man. I am persuaded beyond a shadow of a doubt that this discovery by Dr. Govallo's discovery is genuine. But who could blame the average person today who is bombarded by rip-offs, shams, plain and not-so-plain bull, overstatements, and obfuscation for distrusting everything that appears before her or him. One is often admonished to believe nothing one hears and even less of what one reads. And for good reason!

A person of the 1990's sees very little out there to be optimistic about. But not all is gloom and doom. Good things are happening—we just have a hard time learning what they are. The person ill with cancer is even worse off. Odds are of necessity quoted such as 50% of this or that type cancer patients are alive after 5 years and 25% after 10 years.

This observer has the following action recommendations:

1. Support cancer research;
2. If you believe, as I do, that immunoembryotherapy deserves to at least be studied here to see if it can help people, write to your local representative, congressman or member of parliament and demand to know when it is expected to be available in your country;
3. Buy the book *Immunology of Pregnancy and Cancer* and give it as a present to your internist of oncologist. If you purchased this small publication—you will receive a 50% discount on the book;
4. Help us passing out leaflets and spreading the word. Write to us or call with your ideas.

Defy any medical authority to disprove the underlying theory of immunoembryotherapy as well as the clinical results. If they look hard enough, they will also be able to earn money from it. Encourage any doubters to appear publicly to do so and let them argue the facts. In short—make them check it out! When it is checked out, it is my opinion that this therapy will soon become mainstream.

GLOSSARY

In this glossary, we have tried to include understandable definitions of some of the words which one is most likely to encounter in the world of cancer. We welcome readers' suggestions for additional terms or better explanations. Any reader not encountering here a word or phrase they have read or heard is welcome to contact us.

<u>Antibody</u> - a protein produced by the body's immune system in response to an invader, i.e., an infection, virus or toxic substance. Antibodies are triggered by antigens (see antigens). Infection > antigens > antibodies.

<u>Benign</u> - Not malignant. Many growths such as warts, polyps and moles are usually benign although they may become malignant.

<u>Biopsy</u> - a surgical procedure where a doctor removes tissue from a suspicious growth to determine whether it is malignant or not.

<u>Bone Marrow</u> - the soft, spongy material found inside the cavities of bone.

Breast Examination - Every woman should look for lumps, discharges, or changes each month - for menstruating women at midcycle - for others the same time each month. Charts should be readily available from your physician. If you don't understand how to do it, contact us and we will send you a picture. Doing this test yourself each month costs nothing, so why not do it - you can't lose.

Carcinogens - a cancer-causing agent.

Carcinoma - a malignant tumor originating from epithelial tissues (such as mucous membrane in glands, skin, urinary bladder, nerves and lungs).

CAT Scan - stands for computerized axial tomography. These images are performed by radiology department. The technique uses both x-rays and a computer. There is usually no discomfort associated with this test.

Catheter - a flexible, hollow tube passed into the body to inject or withdraw fluids.

Cells - the basic building blocks of animal and plant tissue. Most patients hear the word connected to the key question of whether the cancer has spread to surrounding tissue, the lymph nodes, or metastasized.

Chemotherapy - the use of drugs to treat cancer. Whether chemotherapy is effective or not depends on the type of cancer and the interaction of the person's organism with the chemotherapy. Chemotherapy can be used alone or in conjunction with surgery and radiation therapy. The drugs used are quite potent and side effects are to be expected. The average cancer patient can expect to go through some form of chemotherapy.

Chromosomes - threadlike structures in the cell nucleus. Humans have 46 chromosomes (23 pairs). Chromosomes are made up of genes which carry genetic information concerning heredity characteristics. One often sees this word in the newspaper connected to genomes and the latest research - genome mapping. It is possible that genome mapping will be very useful one day in cancer research, especially concerning cancers running in families.

Colon - the largest part of the large intestine or bowel. It is 5 to 6 feet long with the last 5 or 6 inches the rectum, which leads outside the body.

Combination Chemotherapy - use of two or more anticancer drugs to treat a patient. Often the effect is somehow stronger when two or more anticancer drugs are used in combination than if they were used sequentially.

Cure - generally refers to elimination of evidence of cancer for a period of 5 years. To the average person, use of the word cure for what may really be a five-year timeout may seem like a misnomer.

Cyst - an abnormal sac in the body containing gas, fluid or a semi-solid substance (have a membrane lining). May or may not be malignant.

DNA - (deoxyribonucleic acid) one of the two nucleic acids found in all cells - the other is RNA (ribonucleic acid). There are many types of DNA including one carrying the genetic message for hereditary characteristics. DNA typing is now even used in criminal cases since each person's is unique.

Etiology - the study of the causes of a disease and how it functions.

Fiber - a component of the diet very significant for reducing the risk of cancer. Foods high in fiber content are vegetables, whole grains and fruits.

Govallo Anticancer Preparation (GAP) - this term refers to the placental extracts and their use discovered and developed by Dr. Valentin I. Govallo. Their history and success are described in his medical book "Immunology of Pregnancy and Cancer" published by Nova Science Publishers in 1992.

Govallo Oncogenic Risk Test - a simple blood test developed by Dr. Valentin I. Govallo to determine malignancy and to predict risk of cancer development.

Hematologist - a doctor who specializes in the blood and blood tissues.

Hodgkin's Disease - a type of cancer which affects the lymphatic and related tissue. Treatment of Hodgkin's Disease has been one of the bright lights of cancer treatments in recent decades. Combination chemotherapy alone or with radiation therapy has been yielding 50-80% cure rates.

Hybridomas - a tumor of hybrid cells used in the production of specific monoclonal antibodies.

Immunoembryotherapy - the term for the cancer therapy developed by Dr. Valentin I. Govallo which utilizes placental extracts (from the afterbirth) to disarm tumors.

Immunologist - a doctor who specializes in the human immunological system. Basically, this is the study of the biological systems within the body which fight off disease. Progress in immunology research is one of the real keys to hopes for significant medical advances in the future.

Immunology - see immunologist.

Immunotherapy - treatment which stimulates the body's own immune system to destroy cancerous cells.

Interferon - a protein our bodies produce regularly whose function is to protect our cells from invasion. Interferon is said to be the first line of defense against attack. Treatment of cancer with interferon has been successful in some cases, but so far the success has been modest.

Lesion - a lump, an abscess or a mass of cells. Can be benign or malignant.

Leukemia - cancers of the blood and circulatory system, usually arising in the bone marrow. Most common of the childhood cancers although far more common in adults.

Melanoma - a skin cancer that often starts as a dark-pigmented mole. Watch all moles for changes. If these are unchecked, they can attack lymph nodes and other organs. It is the deadliest of all skin diseases. Fortunately, the cure rate is now good if caught early. Stay alert if you have moles. It is advisable to stay out of the sun or, if you must, use a strong sunscreen preparation.

Leukocytes - white blood cells produced in the lymphoid organs, such as lymph nodes, spleen, and thymus. Leukocytes are very important for the body's defense against infection.

Lymph Nodes - these are small organs scattering throughout the body and range from the size of a pin to that of a bean. Lymph nodes are important because they are part of the immune system. Often a cancer patient hears or reads a sentence saying whether the lymph nodes were involved or not, which seems to mean to the average patient that the cancer may have begun to spread. Cancer of these organs themselves is called lymphoma. The lymph nodes normally act to filter body impurities.

Lymphoma - cancer arising in the lymph glands or spleen.

Lymphocytes - white blood cells which make up about 22-28 percent of all leukocytes.

Macrophages - scavenger white blood cells which carry away dead cells in the body. The cells are an important part of the body's immunologic defensive mechanism.

Malignant - cancerous (having the property of locally invasive and destructive growth and metastasis).

Mammogram - an x-ray examination of the breast used for cancer detection. Women above 35 years of age should have this test once per year, or at the maximum once every two years. Remember - time counts. The earlier it is detected, the higher the cure rate.

Mastectomy - surgical excision (removal) of the breast. Studies don't seem to show any statistical advantages for radial mastectomy (complete removal) over subcutaneous mastectomy (removal of the tissue but sparing the breast).

Metastasis - spreading of cancerous cells to parts of the body distant from the original site of the cancer. This is a bad word! If you hear it in relation to a cancer of concern to you, it is not a good sign.

Monoclonal Antibodies - an antibody produced by a clone or genetically homogeneous population of hybrid cells.

MRI - Magnetic Resonance Imaging. An imaging technique used in cancer diagnosis among other things.

NCI - National Cancer Institute - the American institute responsible for overseeing cancer research and education. It is located in Bethesda, Maryland.

Neoplasm - a tumor, abnormal growth, or swelling of tissue. It can be either benign or malignant. It is usually malignant.

Nephrologist - a doctor who specializes in diseases of the kidneys.

Neuroblastoma - a tumor of the nervous system.

Oncogenes - cancer genes which may be connected with chromosomal changes causing normal genes to become cancerous.

Oncologist - a medical doctor specializing in the treatment or study of cancer. You can find the nearest one to you by going to your library and looking up medical oncologists in the reference section. If you can't find out, contact us and we will be happy to send you a list.

Pap test - a test to determine changes in the body indicative of cancer. In the case of the cervix, it is diagnostic of cancer (also of pleural [chest] fluid).

Pesticides - probably the source of an enormous amount of cancers. Go organic whenever possible and wash, wash, wash fruit and vegetables prior to consumption.

Placenta - an organ for metabolic interchange between an embryo and the mother. Extracts from the placenta are used for many purposes including drugs and cosmetics. One part was discovered by Dr. Govallo to have an anticancer effect on certain types of cancer.

Plasma Cells - a type of leukocyte which synthesizes circulating antibodies (immunoglobins).

Prostate - the male gland which surrounds the urethra next to the inner wall of the rectum, directly below the bladder. This organ is about the size of a walnut. Second only to lung cancer as the most frequent cancer among American males. 98% occur after age 50. Many prostate cancers respond favorably to hormone treatment. Important that routine rectal digital examination be done each year on men over 40 since in the majority of cases there are no symptoms. When symptoms do occur, they include blood in the urine and painful or burning sensations when urinating.

Radiation Therapy - the treatment of cancer using x-rays and other radiant energy. One of the main three types of current cancer therapy along with surgery and chemotherapy. Radiation therapy almost always results in sizeable doses of radiation reaching noncancerous organs. Side effects can be far reaching. Check with your physician on what to expect (each patient reacts differently so don't rely on the grapevine).

Remission - stopping or slowing down in the symptoms or indicators of cancer. Most people think of remission as a period where the cancer is inactive but could come back at any time.

Sarcoma - cancer that arises in bones and from tissues which connect or lie between organs and the skin. These are usually highly malignant. There are several types. Most sarcomas occur in young people. Survival rates have been increasing in recent years due to new advances in treatment.

Staging - determination of the extent of the cancer. Usually I, II, III, or A, B, C, with IV and D used in some cancers. Each stage can also have subdesignators. The least involvement is I or A.

Toxic reaction - serious side effects or reactions which can be potentially dangerous.

Tumor - an abnormal swelling in the body which serves no useful purpose. They may be cancerous or benign. Tumors start out about the size of a pin. The critical event with tumors occurs when they begin to develop their own blood supplies.

Urologist - a medical doctor who specializes in the treatment and study of the male genitourinary tract and female urinary tract diseases.

Virus - a member of a group of submicroscopic agents infecting humans (and plants). Viruses can divide and multiply only when they feed on a living cell. There are many types of viruses including herpes, human immunodeficiency (HIV), and influenza.

X-ray - a gamma ray used to image the interior of the body. X-rays are important weapons in the diagnosis and treatment of cancer since they can help evaluate the progress of the disease.

REGISTRATION FORM

If you would like to learn of new publications or developments on cancer or cancer immunoembryotherapy, please xerox the form below, fill it out and mail it to us.

**Nova Science Publishers, Inc.
6080 Jericho Turnpike, Suite 207
Commack, New York 11725-2808**

Please keep me informed of new publications on cancer or cancer immunoembryotherapy.

Name: _____
Address: _____
_____
_____
Phone: _____

ISBN 1-56072-107-3